Cure Key

How to Cure from Incurable Diseases

by Spiritual Method (Female & Male)

ISBN-13: 978-1540678171
ISBN-10: 1540678172

CURE KEY

How to Cure from Incurable Diseases

by Spiritual Method

Nothim Assange

ACADEMIC PUPLISHER

Academic Publisher

2016

Copyright

Dedication

To
whom from narrowed his ways...
To
whom lost the Health and wellness.
To
who believes in Creator.
To
who needs a miracle.

If you are in case of disease and illness. And ways narrowed and you LOST methods of healing ... I offer you my individual experience, a wonderful mantra. YOU Will succeed in getting your Health and wellness...

Every sane and specialist, knows very well the importance of the spiritual will and power, in the hope of recovery the healing. Therefore, that our proposed method does not interfere with medical treatment - if any - it supports the medical treatment, and provides introductions objective to heal. But if medical treatment failed, there is no damage while you used our proposal in this book, it is based on the proven spiritual and moral methods of treatment.

My friend reader: You can try to solve your problem, which you have failed to resolve materially, in a condition there should be a will, faith and patience, with benefiting from my experiment.

Note, those texts in this book, were provided by documented referfences. This speech may be new for you and strange ... but there is the opportunity to enter a new world, a future of the Health, wellness and happiness. Whether you're an Atheist or a Believer in the unseen ... I offer you correct advice. I knew a lot of people Try it, AND I tried it personally ... And I succeeded .

Contents

CURE KEY

IF YOU'RE AN ATHEIST

Dear reader:

If you're an atheist ... And you do not see any presence of the Creator of the universe, please note: This is not a book to prove that ... because prove the existence of the Creator needs logical and mentality evidence. THAT is not here, in this book ... BUT The aim of this book is to present only a personal experience You may benefit from them.

WAY PROCESS:

First, decide with yourself, with patience and fortitude, even accomplish the miracle ... That You will be He will succeed to achieve the target.

Note: YOUR faith in divine ability is the foundation for the success of the miracle.

Second: You are preparing to work 40 days in accordance with this method.

Third: start wash at running water (clean water of pipe) or river.

According to the way in which I will explain later

Fourth: You should work at night, after sleeping of family and friends, in order to ensure calm and avoid any ridicule. If you want to do it during the day, try to get a quiet place, preferably on a farm or forest or any quiet and secluded place.

I advise you with fasting during this period of 40 days.

According to the way in which I will explain later

WASHING METHOD:

FIRST, decide to leave all the bad deeds and dirty business; bad business that are causing you discomfort, which make you feel nervous, when you have the feeling upset about those annoying behavior.

SECONDLY, decided - with yourself - to start a new beginning in your life after releasing ... YOU Will be a FRIEND of the Creator ... Who created you ... and HE will help you ... You will be thankful to him.

THIRD: start wash by clean water (water of pipe).

FOURTH:

Wash yourself from the past and clear the last previous malicious acts, by water ... as follows:

THE WAY:

If you washed in the bathroom, or any other ...

- Wash your head and neck first.

- Wash the right side of your body.

- Wash the left side of your body.

- Leave your body dry naturally without drying.

Note:

- You should be directed heartily to the CREATOR before you start panning (washing) ... and feel like you are standing in front of him ... between his hands.

- You must enter the water in possible places of your body.

- Wash your eyes and your nails and the spaces between your fingers

- I would recommend you to start any work with words (with the name of God) ... in a whisper, or in your heart.

IMPORTANT POINT:

A miracle will happen when you get contact with the Creator.

Imagine yourself that you are a man is in a sea, and threatened with drowning… But you do not see anything .. only the sky and the sea ... This sense of danger ... IT WILL OPEN THE GATES OF HEAVEN FOR YOU ...

That time, you will trend towards a lifesaver (THE CREATER) ... This provides conditions, for the descent from heaven jacket rescue.

Note: When Pharaoh and his army, attacked Moses (Prophet Moses) with his group, until they arrived at the edge of the sea ... Hard Situation: Nothing only the sea and the army of Pharaoh ... Moses's group had a tension ... And his people began shouting against him (Prophet Moses) …

They said: Where is the Lord, O Moses ... Where is your Lord? … This is Pharaoh and his killer army is coming. AND This is the sea ...

O Moses! ... YOU 've deceived us ... Pharaoh will kill us all ... And ONE will not save us ...

MOSES SAID: I trust my Lord

Pharaoh's army arrived to Moses ... and everyone confused. And death became a fact and very near.

.. SUDDENLY THE SEA WAS SPLITED...

Moses and his people ran to the other side ...

Pharaoh's army ran behind them. But they were sinking

Moses and his people were survived.

DEAR: BE LIKE DROWNING IN A SEA ... DO NOT SEE ONLY THE CREATOR ... THEN THE MIRACLE WILL COME.

FASTING METHOD:

The basic idea of fasting, isolation of the mind from the physical, materialist noise, and in order to find a suitable atmosphere for spiritual starting point. So I enclosed another book with this book, entitled "Fasting and salvation" for additional information. But I will write for you, here, the important things, that are required and enough, as follows:

First, the purpose of fasting is to draw closer to the Creator.

Second: define a particular time, to abide by it (fasting) every day.

Third, repeat this fortieth day.

Fourth, throughout this period, eating vegetarian food.

Fifth: to avoid the meat of animals and its oil, except fish.

Sixth: I recommend to determine some hours in the daytime, you be in fast during this hours, from all food and drink, based on your ability and willingness.

O God, O sufficient to the isolated and weak

and Protector against terrifying affairs!

Offenses have isolated me, so there is none to be my companion.

I am too weak for Thy wrath and there is none to strengthen me.

I have approached the terror of meeting Thee

and there is none to still my fear.

Who can make me secure from Thee when Thou hast filled me with terror?

Who can come to my aid

when Thou hast isolated me?

Who can strengthen me when Thou hast weakened me?

None can grant sanctuary to a vassal, my God, but a lord,

none can give security to one dominated but a dominator,

none can aid him from whom demands are made but a demander.

In Thy hand, my God, is the thread
of all that,

in Thee the place of escape and
flight,

so bless Prophets,

give sanctuary to me in my flight,

and grant my request!

O God, if Thou should turn Thy
generous face away from me,

withhold from me Thy immense
bounty,

forbid me Thy provision,

or cut off from me Thy thread,

I will find no way to anything of
my hope other than Thee

nor be given power over what is
with Thee through another's aid,

for I am Thy servant and in Thy
grasp; my forelock is in Thy hand.

I have no command along with Thy
command.

Accomplished is Thy judgement of
me,

just Thy decree for me!'

I have not the strength to emerge
from Thy authority

nor am I able to step outside Thy power.

I cannot win Thy inclination,

arrive at Thy good pleasure,

or attain what is with Thee except through obeying Thee and through the bounty of Thy mercy.

O God, I rise in the morning and enter into evening

as Thy lowly slave.

I own no profit and loss for myself except through Thee.

I witness to that over myself

and I confess to the frailty of my strength and the paucity of my strata-gems.

So accomplish what Thou hast promised me

and complete for me what Thou hast given me,

for I am Thy slave, miserable, abased, frail, distressed, vile,

despised, poor, fearful, and seeking sanctuary!

O God, bless Prophets

and let me not forget to remember Thee in what Thou hast done for me, be heedless of Thy beneficence in Thy trying me,

or despair of Thy response to me, though it keeps me waiting,

whether I be in prosperity or adversity,

hardship or ease,

well-being or affliction,

misery or comfort,

wealth or distress,

poverty or riches!

O God, bless Prophets,

make me laud Thee, extol Thee,

and praise Thee in all my states

so that I rejoice not over what Thou
gives' me of this world

nor sorrow over that of it which
Thou withhold from me!

Impart reverential fear of Thee to
my heart,

employ my body in that which
Thou accept from me,

and divert my soul through obedience to Thee from all that enters upon
me,

so that I love nothing that dis-
pleases Thee and become displeased
at nothing that pleases Thee!

O God, bless Prophets,

empty my heart for Thy love,

occupy it with remembering Thee,

animate it with fear of Thee and
quaking before Thee,

strengthen it with beseeching Thee,

incline it to Thy obedience,

set it running in the path most be-
loved to Thee,

and subdue it through desire for what is with Thee all the days of my life!

Let my provision in this world be reverential fear of Thee,

my journey be toward Thy mercy,

and my entrance be into Thy good pleasure!

Appoint for me a lodging in Thy Garden,

give me strength to bear everything that pleases Thee,

make me flee to Thee

and desire what is with Thee,

clothe my heart in estrangement from the evil among Thy creatures,

and give me intimacy with Thee,

Thy friends, and those who obey Thee!

Assign to no wicked person or un-believer a kindness toward me

or a hand that obliges me,

nor to me a need for one of them!

Rather make the stillness of my heart, the comfort of my soul,

my independence and my suffi-ciency

lie in Thee and the best of Thy creatures!

O God, bless Prophets,

make me their comrade,

make me their helper,

and oblige me with yearning for Thee

and doing for Thee What Thou love and approve!

Thou art powerful over everything

and that is easy for Thee.

Take a rest, and I suggest that you to wash the same way, and then go to the second prayer of supplication. This was repeated for 40 days.

My God, let not my enemy gloat
over me

and torment not my dear kinsman
or friend through me!

My God, of Thy glances, give me
one glance,

and thereby remove from me that
by which Thou hast afflicted me

and return me to the best of Thy
customs with me!

Respond to my supplication

and the supplication of him who devotes his supplication sincerely to Thee,

for my power has become frail,

my stratagems few,

my situation severe,

and I despair of what is with Thy creatures,

so nothing remains for me but hope in Thee!

My God, surely Thy power to remove that in which I dwell

is like Thy power in that with which Thou hast afflicted me!

And surely the remembrance of Thy acts of kindliness comforts me

and hope in Thy showing favor and Thy bounty strengthens me,

for I have not been without Thy favor ever

since Thou created me.

And Thou, my God, art my place of flight, my asylum,

my protector, my defender,

the loving toward me, the compassionate,

and the guarantor of my provision.

In Thy decree lay what has settled
upon me

and in Thy knowledge that to
which I have come home.

So, my Patron and Master, place

within that which Thou hast or-
dained, decreed, and made
unavoidable for me,

my well-being and that wherein lies
my soundness

and my deliverance from that in
which I am!

I hope for none to repel this other than Thee, and I rely in it only upon Thee.

O Possessor of majesty and munificence, be with my best opinion of Thee!

Have mercy upon my frailty and the paucity of my stratagems,

remove my distress,

grant my supplication,

ease me from my stumble,

and show kindness to me in that

and to everyone who supplicates Thee!

My Master, thou hast commanded me to supplicate

and undertaken to respond,

and Thy promise is the truth in which there is no failing, nor any change.

So bless all prophets and your servant,

and the pure, the Folk of his House,

and help me,

surely Thou art the help of him who has no help

and the stronghold of him who has no stronghold,

while I am the distressed

the response to whom and the removal of evil from whom Thou hast made obligatory!

So respond to me, remove my concern,

relieve my gloom,

return my state to the best it has been,

and repay me not according to what I deserve,

but according to Thy mercy which embraces all things,

O Possessor of majesty and munifi-cence!

Bless all prophets and your servant,

and the pure, the Folk of his House,

hear, and respond, O All-mighty!

- NOTES:
- Read this supplication or prayer forty times.
- Be sure to isolation yourself from any ideas and others when you are reading,
- Try to gently prays to the Creator
- Be sure to get a miracle from the Creator
- HE will help you in the fastest time... Trust Him Absolutely Confident

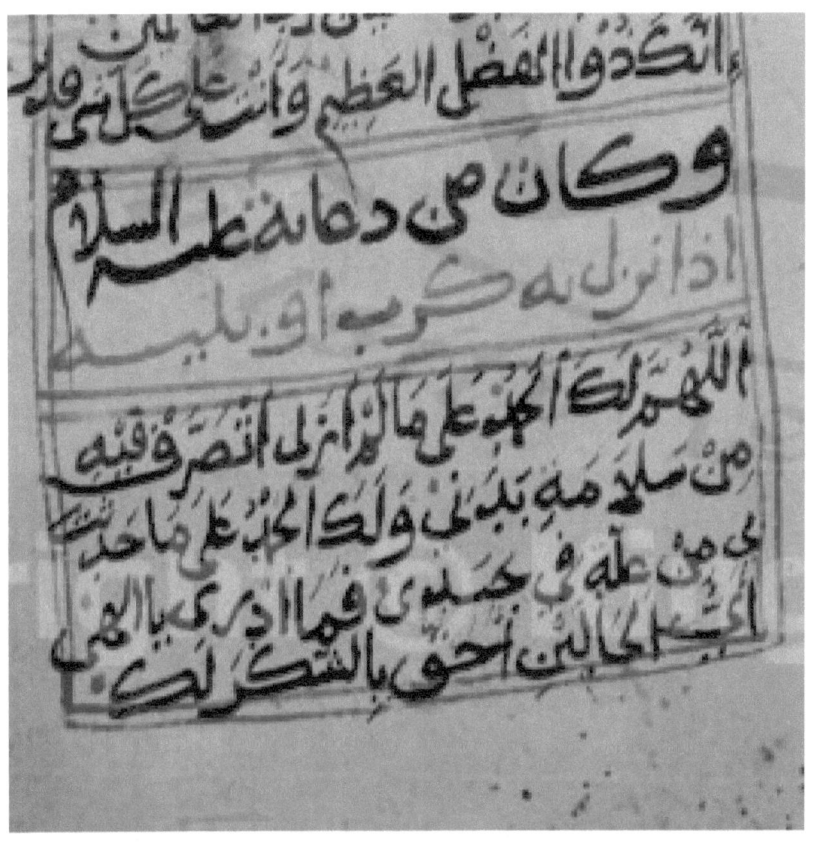

وأيُّ الوقتين أولى بأنْ هذَلك أوقّتُ
الضُّحى هاتاني فيها طَبَقاتِ رِزْقِكَ
وتُطمني فيها أنعامَ رضاتِكَ
و وصلكَ وقوّني معها على ما
وفقتني له من طاعتِكَ أم وقت
العلّةِ التي مخصني بها والنِّعَمِ التي
أحفني بها عفوها لاتعمل على طهري
من الخطايا وتُطهر الماء انغسل فيه
من الشّهات ونفيها لتأول التّوبه
وتذكّرا المحو الجوية بقدم نبرآتمعه وفي
خلال ذلك ما كتب لي الكاتبان
من زكي الأعمال ملا قلبه فكرفيه
ولا لسان نطق به ولا جارحه تكلفه
بل إفضالا منكَ عليّ وإحسانا من

صنيعك الى فضل على محمد وآله

وحبب الى ما رضيت لى وتسرط

ما أحللت وطهرني من دنس

ما أسلفت وامح عني شر ما قد مت

وأو جهني خلاوه العافيه و

أذقني برد السلامه وأجعل خرجي

عن علتي الى عفوك ومتحولي عن

صرعتي الى تجاوزك وخلاصي من

كربي الى روحك وسلامتي من

هذه النله في الى فرجك انك

المفضل بالاحسان المطول بالامتنان

الوهاب الكريم ذو الجلال والاكرام

وكان من دعايه عليه السلام

MY FRIEND THE READER ..

My friend the reader ...Thank you for your interest with this book. There is a printed copy and audio at Amazon site. Please do not hesitate to send your feedback and messages to me at the address:drnadhim@gmail.com

Note: We have added the book of "Fasting and salvation" with this book, for additional information.

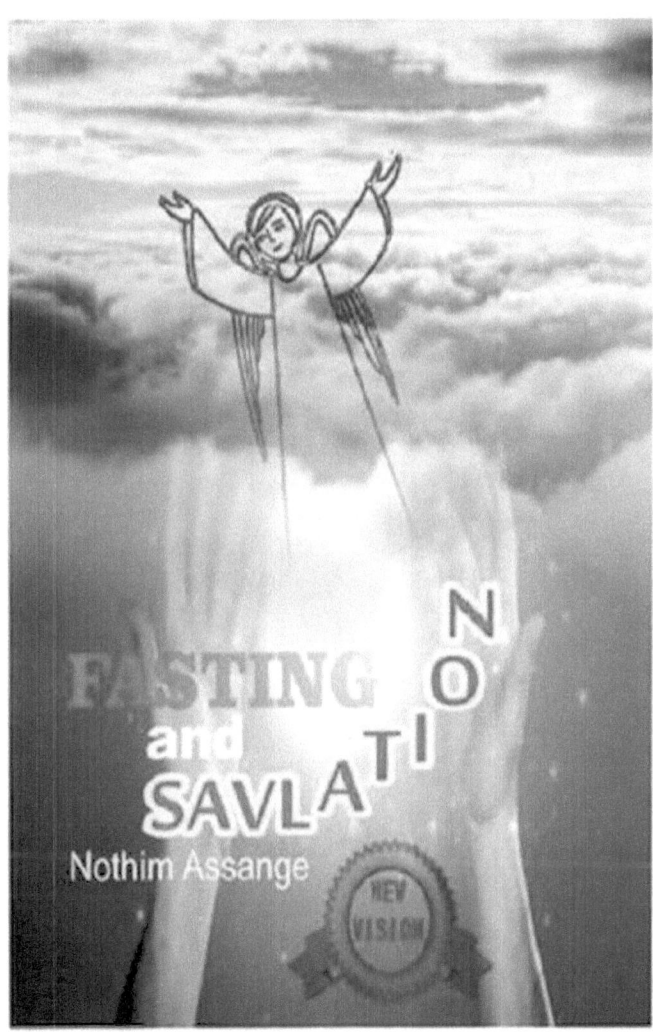

FASTING and SAVLATION

Nothim Assange

NEW VISION

Fasting and Salvation

Buddhism, Hinduism, Judaism, Christianity and Islam,

with a new vision

ISBN-13: 978-1535020466

ISBN-10: 1535020466

Fasting And Salvation

Buddhism, Hinduism, Judaism, Christianity and Islam, with a new vision

Nothim Assange

2016

Second Printing: 2016

ISBN-13: 978-1535020466

ISBN-10: 1535020466

drnadhim@gmail.com

Printed in the United States.

Dedication

To whom

  feel the tragedy of mankind

  ...

To whom

  feel alienated of human

  ....

To whom

  feel the greatness of human.....

Contents

Acknowledgements

I would like to thank my family...

without whose help this book would never have been completed.

Thank you...

for your patience and guidance.

Foreword

I THINK THAT something has been missing from researchers; An integrated project leads the universe. The concept of the divine project and the divine planning for the development of the universe are Important elements for understanding the cause of human existence and his career and his goals.

The talk about fasting leads us to talk about the moral and spertitual chances of human and his ability, how we are integrating? why we are integrating? Is it possible for us? And what is the savlation..?

IN OTHER WORDS: if we believe that there are higher planning for the development of the universe and the integration of human, it is possible to understand the chance for integration morally. Fasting is an opportunity for integration, divine project support that and he provides a schedule and equips us with energies and conditions.

In this book, a wide and impartial discussion of the cosmic and human integration, Author has informed the subject Capacity. He did not care about the religious vision only, he interested in the material and the secular and Marxist ideology, but the topic needs to be a wider study as well as to reflect on the ultimate goal of this integration, not only from the religious side but also by the physical and secular trend, especially the Marxist trend and the intellectual side of the capitalist economic.

FOR THE FIRST TIME, gets connection between religious and material thought, was reached a common point, a chance of salvation. Also, the book includes a new link between the scattered religious concepts, the writer envisions for the divine project and human fate, which will end to a happy future, which is accelerating the integration, until we meet with other worlds, absent from us now.

We hope that my dear reader will have a broad chest with us.

Introduction

Before that, we need to understand the big issue; the broad concept of human existence, it is necessary to produce a new understanding, is not a traditional. It is an issue of integration and overall development of the universe and humanity. So we have dedicated the first chapter to him.

So were the order of the chapters are as follows:

Chapter 1: Fasting.

Chapter 2: Integration.

Chapter 3: A new Vision.

CHAPTER ONE: INCLUDE the subject; Fasting of Buddhist, Jews, Muslims, Christians, Fasting of other religions and Other types of Fasting. The exposure briefly, for the attention of the reader and openness to other forms of fasting, outside his religion and his group, because the biggest problem is the narrow-mindedness and intolerance, and religious suspicion entitlement without the other, and the manipulation of the believer himself only. Without paying attention to the worship vary from one place to another, and it's a set of movements, nothing more, does not mean anything no matter what their shape, but the important thing is who order them, you ordered by the Director of the universe ..?

Or ordered by the Director of the temple ..? Or ordered by Sheikh Mosque ..? Or ordered by the priest and the priest and the rabbi ..? Or in other words: Do we implement the worship of obedience who created us, or to serve the religious group or sect or party ..?

I find it necessary - here - to refer to the Important notes about worship, as follows:

FIRST, THE SHAPE and the way is not important, if they do not prove it, according to divine orders, and learned that causes our conviction and confidence, that what we do is from the Creator.

SECOND: Why Do I Do This ..? For their relationship and friendship with The Master Of The Universe ..? Or for their friendship and the relationship with the priest or Sheikh or priest or rabbi ..?

THE SECOND CHAPTER of this book is concerned with the subject known as an salvation, but I looked at the subject from another angle, the basis of my understanding of the subject of salvation is based on faith in the willingness of the existence and humanity towards integration, and this based on the support of metaphysical force, making verification of salvation possible, but inevitable. And salvation is in this world, not only in the afterlife. I have a new idea of salvation: for moral and spiritual integrity of humanity after a certain time, resulting in a system socially fair, but not as in Marxism, that this system fair Advanced spiritually, morally, and produces a society happy and perfect.

CHAPTER 3 of this book introduce the new vision for fasting and salvation, and their relationship to integration, and project divine.

Sky has worked to raise us beings to the top, to the level of soul world, but we are trying - always - withdrawal heaven to earth, because of our physical thinking. So Moses, Jesus, Buddha, Mohammed and 124000 a messenger came from heaven, to lift us but we tried to draw them down. Thy tried to open our minds to God and the unseen, but we closed the door with his face

.Unfortunately, humans foiled the efforts of Prophets and Messengers, and instead to live with them, and let us go up, we tried to draw them into the mud and earth, we made them gods of materialists, and idols.

I think, that Marxism, material and secular, are intellectual attempts to save mankind, and to find a solution to our problems, but it is not interested in the spiritual and moral side of our human and considered physical assets only, so it is failed to achieve the dream, as well as caused additional problems for us. Because of the adoption of the authorities and the governments of these physical theories, and the exclusion of moral treatises.

Dear reader ..

When the researcher to review the concept of salvation in religious books, does not find - often - just nonsense and chatter, does not work ..!

This nonsense that we find, not from God, it's illusion-making by the departments of religion, and most of these preachers, they are losers scientifically and academically, who are unemployed, worked in the field of religion, taking advantage of our passion and our kindness..! So one should be careful in dealing with this serious matter, do not think that the issue of faith secondary and trivial ..

This problem we are trying to exposure it, logically, in the third chapter, because we are part of a divine project and his plan, and each of us has the mission and work in this project. The person is responsible to the orders of THE GOD, and this responsibility will be in accordance with real information, and have the foundation of science, based on what was brought by the messagers and prophets, is not enough to talk about this is in the imagination of conjecture.

Methodology Of This Book

THE AUTHOR does not see the possibility of detail of the evidence and proofs and it may be lost main objective of the book and makes it boring, so we used appropriate scientific methodology is based on the An Inductive Logic ; it is a system of evidential support that extends deductive logic to less-than-certain inferences.

Practically, we should read the texts, literature and publications of religious or sectarian groups,then try to extract common elements, that help us to get a full picture about that intellectual or ideological direction of groups.

Fig. 1 showed this simulation of methodology

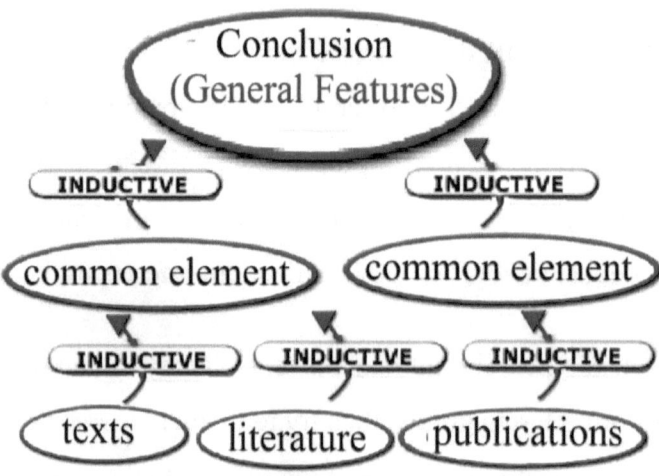

Fig. 1 Simulation of book methodology.

Chapter 1: Fasting

THE FASTING is a wide concept of human's willing to resistance of his material requirements, so may be we can classify it as:

(1) Abstinence or Chastity for a specified period.

(2) Reduction from some or all food, drink, or both, for a period of time.

(3) Refrain from any king's authority and power except the real king; It is a moral spiritual fasting, Its importance in the development of the individual powers and society integration , It will be detailed later in this book.[1]

We can talk about the types of fasting, according to conventional religions as follows:

(1) Fasting of Buddhist

(2) Fasting of Jews.

(3) Fasting of Muslims.

(4) Fasting of Christians

---

[1]This is a moral theme, I could not go into it now, for lack of time, but will write about later.

(5) Fasting of other religions

(6) Refrain from food or hunger strike, as refrain from food of prisoners.

(7) The strike against life (suicide).

Note: The order of religions in this book, it may be due to technical requirements or for reasons of history appearing within human history.

Fasting Of Christian

FASTING IN CHRISTIAN worship and submission to the Lord, and there is no specific date for fasting when Christians. Church tradition has said before fasting forty days of the Easter holiday, then it increased to six weeks of what was called the biggest fasting.

The text in the Bible, there is no static text of this fasting, and schedule differs from year to year. At the foundation it prevents eating animal meat and dairy products and their derivatives, but it is up to the church.

Russian Church prohibits eating meat and fish, the Catholic Church in England, followed allowed to eat meat and fish in the days of fasting, but in just a few days, Wednesday and Friday and Holy Thursday. The Coptic Orthodox Faismon in many days, and abstain from meat and dairy, while allowing eating fish now.

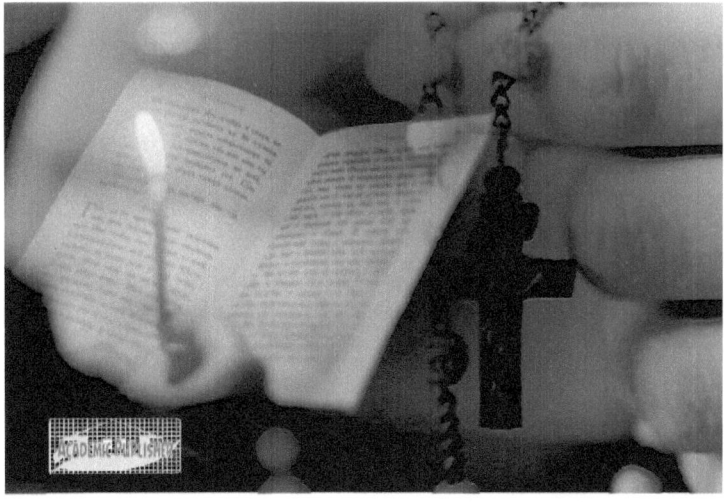

Period Of Fasting

According to a number of Christian sources; there is not a set period of time, that makes Christian fasting lawful. In Bible times, fasts were generally one day in length. Judges 20:26 says;

"Then all the sons of Israel and all the people went up and came to Bethel and wept; thus they remained there before the LORD and fasted that day until evening. And they offered burnt offerings and peace offerings before the LORD."

Occasionally, fasts in Bible times were three days (Esther 4:16)

"Go, gather all the Jews to be found in Susa, and hold a fast on my behalf, and do not eat or drink for three days, night or day. I and my young women will also fast as you do. Then I will go to the king, though it is against the law, and if I perish, I perish."

Or even seven days as in (1 Samuel 31:13). The text is:

"And they took their bones and buried them under the tamarisk tree in Jabesh and fasted seven days."

And on three occasions, fasts lasted 40 days:

(1) Moses receiving the 10 Commandments (Exodus 34:28). The text is:

"So he was there with the Lord forty days and forty nights. He neither ate bread nor drank water. And he wrote on the tablets the words of the covenant, the Ten Commandments."

(2) Elijah encountering God (1 Kings 19:8). The text is:

"And he arose and ate and drank, and went in the strength of that food forty days and forty nights to Horeb, the mount of God."

(3) Jesus being tempted in the wilderness (Matthew 4). The text is:

"Then Jesus was led up by the Spirit into the wilderness to be tempted by the devil. 2 And after fasting forty days and forty nights, he was hungry."

The practice of regular fasting as normal Christian behavior was taught by Jesus; (Mt. 6:16–17, 9:15). The text is:

"Moreover, when you fast, do not be like the hypocrites, with a sad countenance. For they disfigure their faces that they may appear to men to be fasting. Assuredly, I say to you, they have their reward. But you, when you fast, anoint your head and wash your face,

Fasting Of Jews

FASTING FOR JEWS linked to certain occasions and days, and express forgiveness and sin more of it is linked to specific deadlines. Famous days that Jews may do are;

Day of Atonement: it is fast Twenty-five continuous hours. It begins before sunset at about quarter-hour and end after sunset quarter of an hour, from the second day.

They fasted on the anniversary of the demolition of the Temple of Solomon, and fasted on the day of the death of God's prophet Moses, as well as three weeks of fasting and mourning by the Romans in the demolition of the temple and took Jerusalem from the seventeenth of July until the ninth of August, As fast days before the war and fighting, and young man fast on his wedding, and the day his father's death.

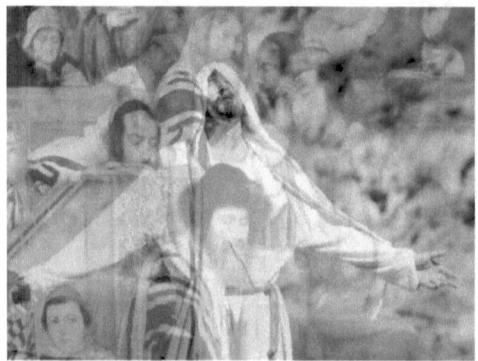

Fasting Of Muslims

FASTING FOR MUSLIMS is to refrain from eating, drinking, sexual intercourse, lying, and other matters. And begin fasting from morning (dawn) until sunset. Muslims fast in the month is called Sha-har Ramadan. Fasting begins at the sighting of the moon at the beginning of its appearance.

The schedule varies annually, according to the solar calendar, But it fixed in accordance with the lunar calendar. Muslims fast more days out of Ramadan, for example; fasting on the day of Arafah and every Monday and Thursday of each week.

Day of 'Arafah is the greatest day of Hajj for Muslims, and the millions of Muslims gather in a particular valley. It is an important day and they have a sacred.

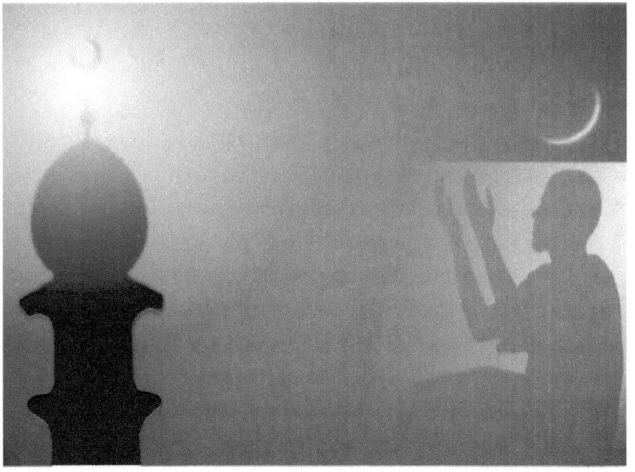

Fasting For Buddhism

BUDDHISM IS FAMOUS in Asia, it has emerged in the fifth century BC, Founded "Buddha" means "an alert man" , also nicknamed "Skamouni" which means retreat, and originated in northern India, and gradually spread across Asia, Tibet and Sri Lanka, and then to China, Mongolia, Korea and Japan, and then split into two illuminated "Theravada" and "Mahayana".

Fasting in Buddhism from sunrise to sunset, in four days of the lunar month are "first, IX, XV, and the twenty-second", and they call it "Alliopomana days", the days of fasting which prohibits practicing any work, even food preparation, for it is those who fast food before sunrise.

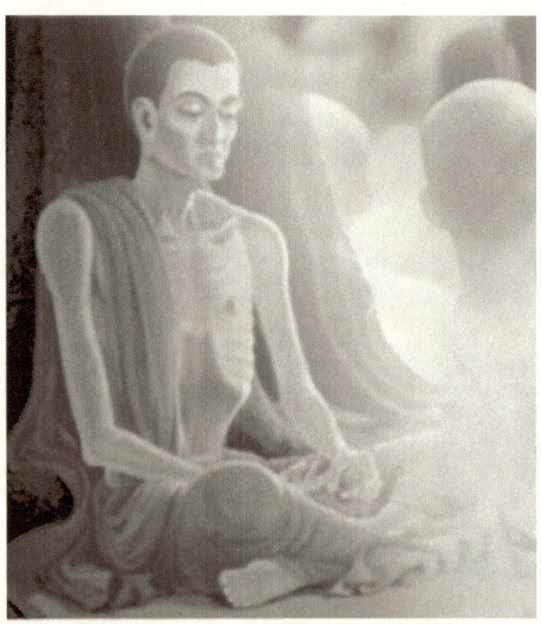

Buddhists regard the fast way to cleanse the human self, and successful tool to liberate the human mind from the illusions and

myths. Buddhism and some of the teams that live in the Tibet Autonomous Region, in the context of fasting and spiritual exercises for the sport of yoga. Fasting they generate internal energy that helps the soul to restrain its desires and ambitions and achieve tranquility and serenity mental. Priests fast extra days and they confess their sins in a whisper.

Buddhist doctrine centered around three things called "Three Jewels" ; First, faith in Buddha as a teacher informed the Buddhist doctrine, The second is the faith to "Dharma", the teachings of the Buddha are called the "truth" in the text of the "Sutra", Third Buddhist community

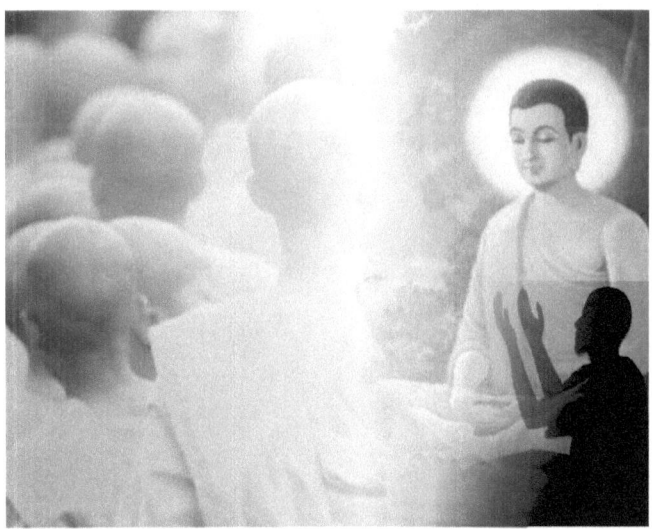

Fasting of Hindus:

HINDUS them ritual fasting, vary depending on The individual God. They are present in southern India, and fasted from sunrise to west, allowing for them to drink liquids only, in the northern areas are allowed to eat fruit and milk only.

They have special fasting called the Fasting of Seasons, they shall refrain in it, of eating from sunrise to sunset, for nine days, a quarterly, it is strange ritual fasting.

Hindu person fasts according to the orders of his God, and they have more than God, who follows God called Shiva fasts Monday, and who follows the god called Vishnu fasts on Thursday. In general, the Hindus in their fast abstain from eating meat.

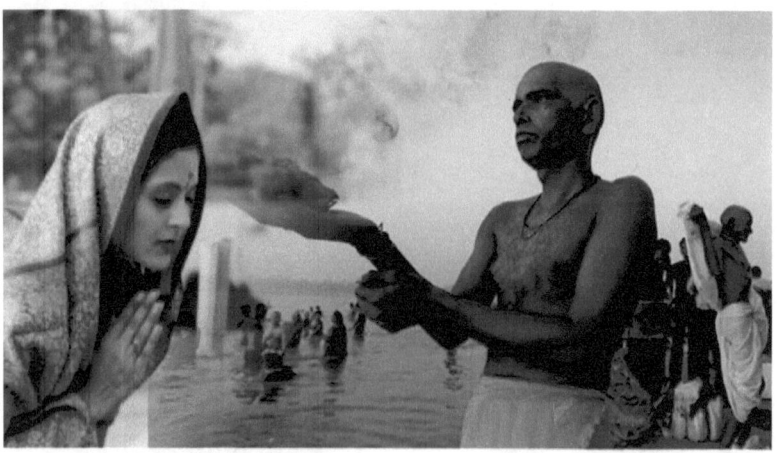

A hunger strike

Is A Way of non-violent resistance or expression in which partic-ipants fast as an act of political protest, or to produce feelings of guilt in oppressor, usually with the objective to achieve a goal, such as achieving justice. Most hunger strikers will take liquids only, but not solid food.

Why it was considered by the author as some kind of fasting..? We can sa; because we look to fast from psychological motives angle. The reasons driving for man to rebel against him self or injustice of others. Surely oppression may be internal by ourselves or by an others and governments.

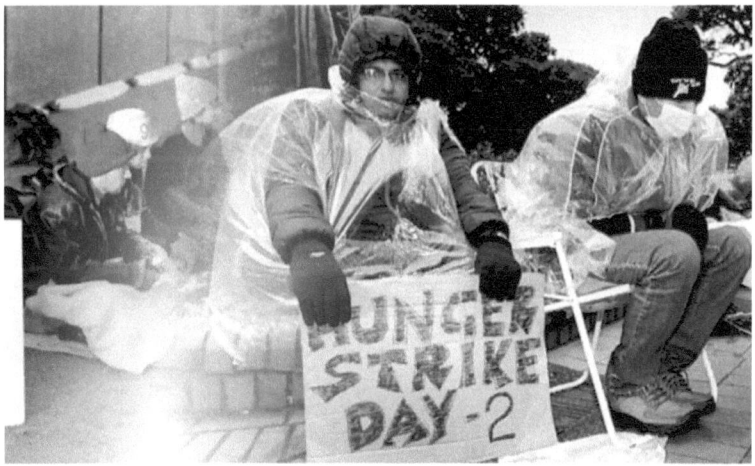

And we can understand fasting as a challenge; challenge against ourselves and our weakness. The prisoner wants to exceed the insult and humiliation, exceeds the internal weaknesses and psychological, and it strengthens its potential in the face of injustice and unjust. He wants to prove that; he is human and has a dignity and value. This is the true philosophy of fasting. The fasting person is trying to triumph over himself and his weakness and strengthens the spiritual and moral potential.

Gandhi has practical application to fast kinetic, aimed at societal integration and the challenge of the big powers. Gandhi has scored brilliant and bright pages in the book of human history. It's peaceful resistance against injustice and domination, sectarianism and racism.

Gandhism is a sum of ideas of that describes the inspiration, vision and the life work of Gandhi. It is particularly associated with his contributions to the idea of nonviolent resistance and sometimes also called civil resistance. The two pillars of "Gandhism" were truth and non-violence.

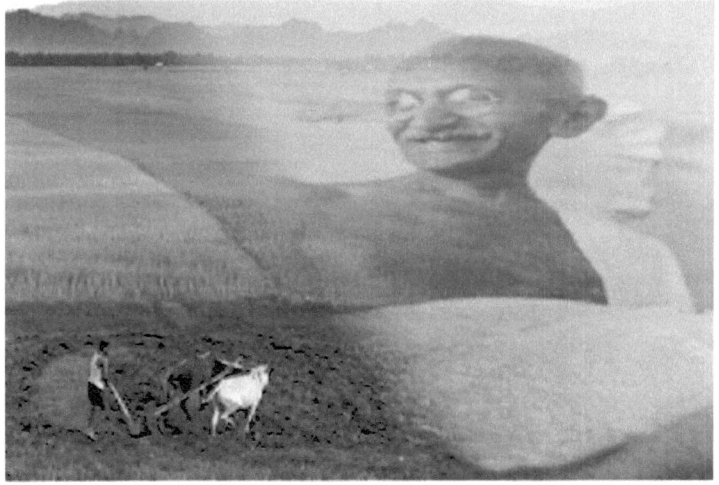

The term "Gandhism" also encompasses what Gandhi's ideas, words and actions mean to people around the world, and how they used them for guidance in building their own future. Gandhism also permeates into the realm of the individual human being, non-political and non-social. A Gandhian can mean either an individual who follows, or a specific philosophy which is attributed to, Gandhism.

Professor Ramjee Singh has called Gandhi a bodhisattva (bodhisattva is the Sanskrit term for anyone who, motivated by great compassion, has generated bodhicitta, which is a spontaneous wish to attain buddhahood for the benefit of all sentient beings. Bodhisattvas are a popular subject in Buddhist art of the twentieth century).[1]

Suicide

Sometimes we find the right solution, or we choose the wrong way. Wrong decision when we decide to escape from life and its challenges because of a feeling of weakness and defeat The person refrain from eating of life and drinking fresh air ..!

We are against suicide but the reason is the sense of injustice internal or external, from ourselves or from others or unjust authority. This falls within our understanding of Fasting but Suicide is a bad type, because of sabotage and not integration.

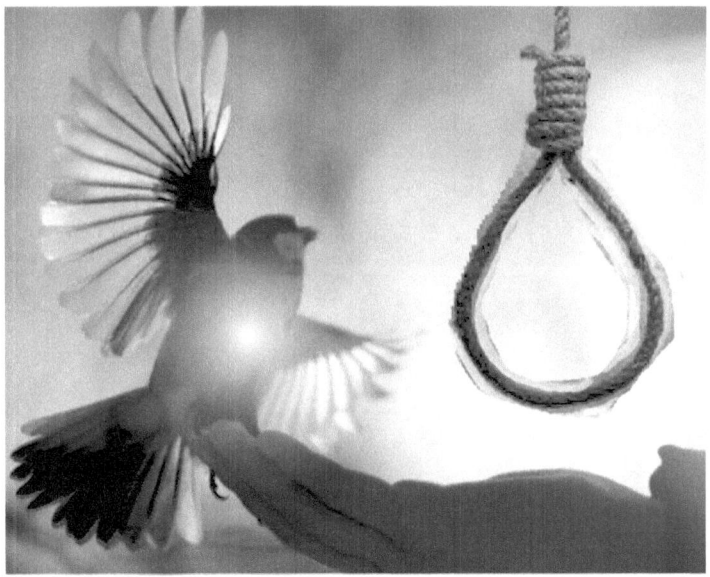

Heaven and humanity rejects this weakness and defeatism Suicide is the act of intentionally causing one's own death. Risk factors include mental illness such as depression, bipolar disorder,

Schizophrenia, personality disorders, alcoholism, or drug abuse. Others are impulsive acts due to stress such as from financial difficulties, troubles with relationships, or bullying. Those who have previously attempted suicide are at high risk of future attempts. Suicide prevention efforts include limiting access to method of suicide such as firearms and poisons, treating mental illness and drug misuse, proper media reporting of suicide, and improving economic conditions. Although crisis hotlines are common, there is little evidence for their effectiveness.[2-6]

These views are not comprehensive and not a full general, because the suicides happened in the case of the face at the jail or war; for example, suicides obtained by the Nazi Germans and Japanese officers committed suicide. Today we have a large proportion of suicides .. Why ..? It can be explained because of the physical pressures and economic pressures and societal injustice, but the first reason is the weakness of the individual's moral.

May be he strengthens him self by cut off his life, and rejects life and injustice. If a person has a spiritual and moral force, he is not going to commit suicide, he remains to resist peacefully instead of escape.

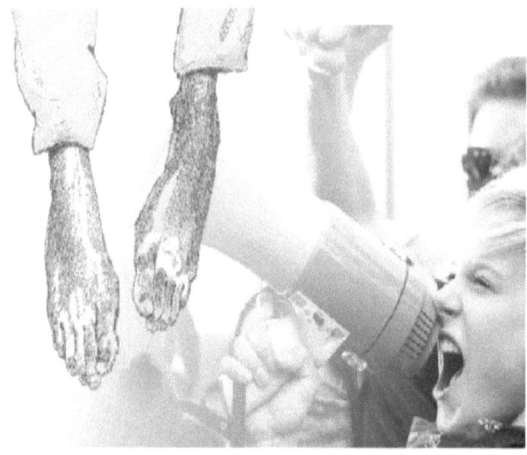

On the other hand, that the struggle against the dictatorship may cause death. Do you struggle suicide ..? Or is fasting for life with the dictator, as well as resistance to occupation might produce death .. .. Is this a suicide? Or is it the fast life ruled by the occupier ..?

Therefore, we mentioned that we are talking about fasting. Refrain from life as possible, if life was caused humiliation and contempt. But suicide at home is an act of cowards, and if the ruling is injustice, we have to fight for change and reform, and we give our lives in exchange for salvation, that Christ has done and Guevara and Gandhi and others, they have sacrificed for mankind ..

Trying To Understand

THE PROBLEM IS the loss of a sense of human unity, any way, the enemy is also human also, it is our duty to pass on to him our understanding in any way. This happened by the Prophet Ibrahim when he faced the government and the temple, thus Moses was when he faced the Pharaoh, thus, Jesus was when he faced the oppressors, and so it was the Prophet Muhammad when confronted with the Government of the Hijaz and Quraish, so it is the Gandhi way in the face of the international community and injustice.

This is an attempt to go deeper in the philosophy of fasting; the reasons that drive human resistance to internal and external pressur. That the individual always tries to integration, as well as human society is moving towards integration, as well as the entire assets seeks integration, and Integration gradual down for salvation.

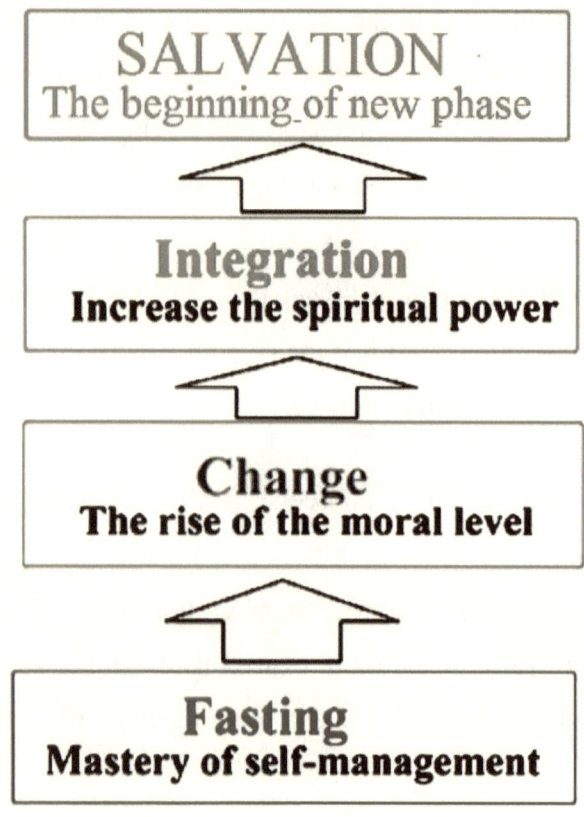

Fig. (2) The steps of Integration.

Salvation can understand it is a line change and we can discuss a new understanding, different from the traditional understanding of the churches and temples, broader and deeper understanding. Why..? you can say: That salvation determines the future of the universe and human rights and his futur.

This is the most important goal of the author, I hope that the reader excuse me, and sought his mind with me, and divest himself of his affiliation, to become clearer the picture, I do not mean to impose the doctrine, but I try to be neutral, and launched into reflection on our reality and our future.

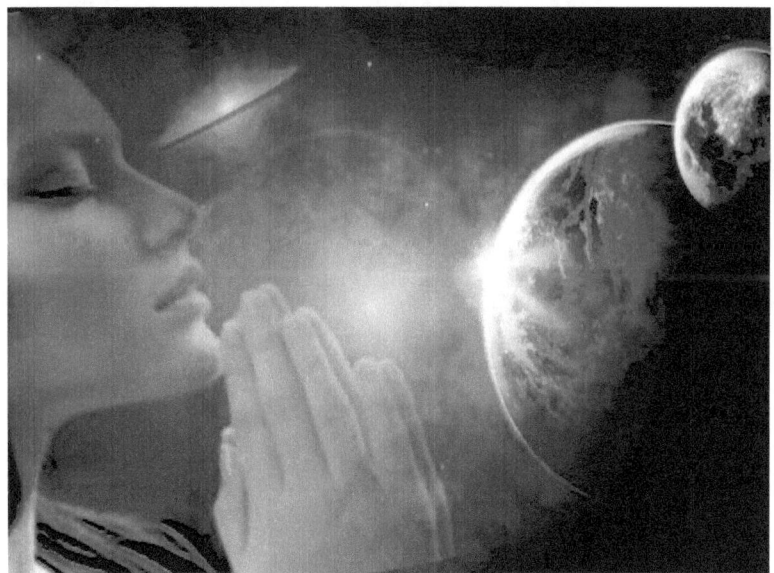

A New Vision

It seems that a significant effect of fasting is clear and uncertain, but this will effect the moral needs of the individual, that will is reasoned that fasting and nothing else. I mean; that does not have to fast because of belonging to a group and it is intended to uphold the value of the group or because a political goal of fasting or regional.

I mean; not to be fasting for their financial objectives, such as slimming and weight reduction. Despite the proven positive health impact of fasting but fasting has health effect the most important spiritual and mental In Islam said (Somo Tashoa). Muslims understand this talk of prophetic, it refers to physical health, this is true, but there is a better understanding; it is fast in order to wake up.

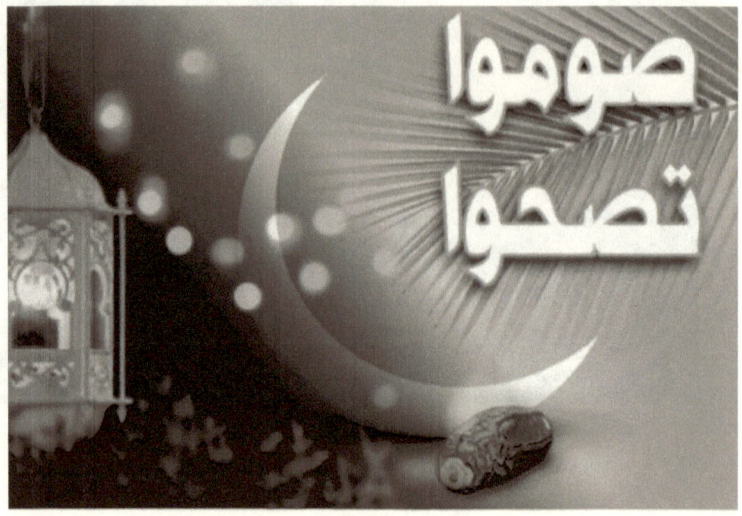

Fast when healthy minds and vigilance and it supports this meaning the verse says:

O you who believe! Observing As-Saum (the fasting) is prescribed for you as it was prescribed for those before you, that you may become Al-Muttaqun (the pious - see V.2:2).

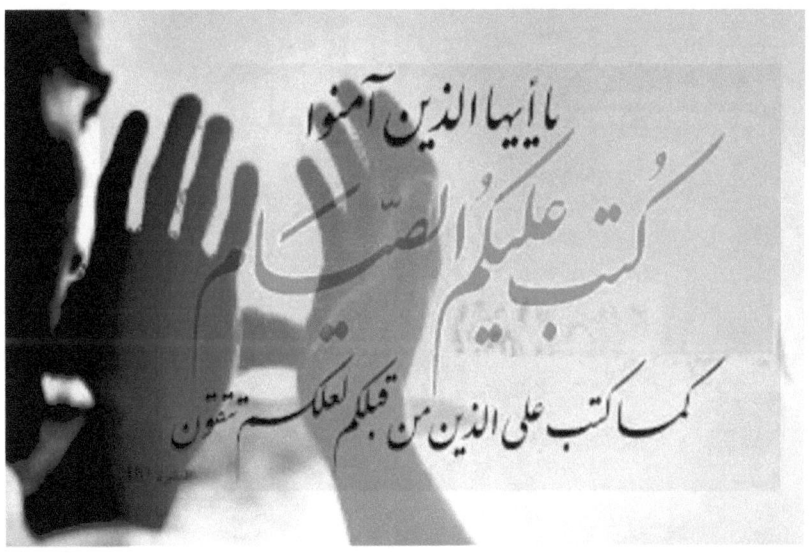

Because the act of piety spiritual and mental and understanding correctly in both cases but the meaning of (Somo Tasheo), it is to get the sense of awakening and vigilance. This includes all religions and not only Muslims,

So Atheists said; that religion is the opium of the people, because the clerics do not like the vigilance of the people for economic reasons, except for a few of them, with my respect to the clergy-loving peoples and peace spiritual, mental and integration.

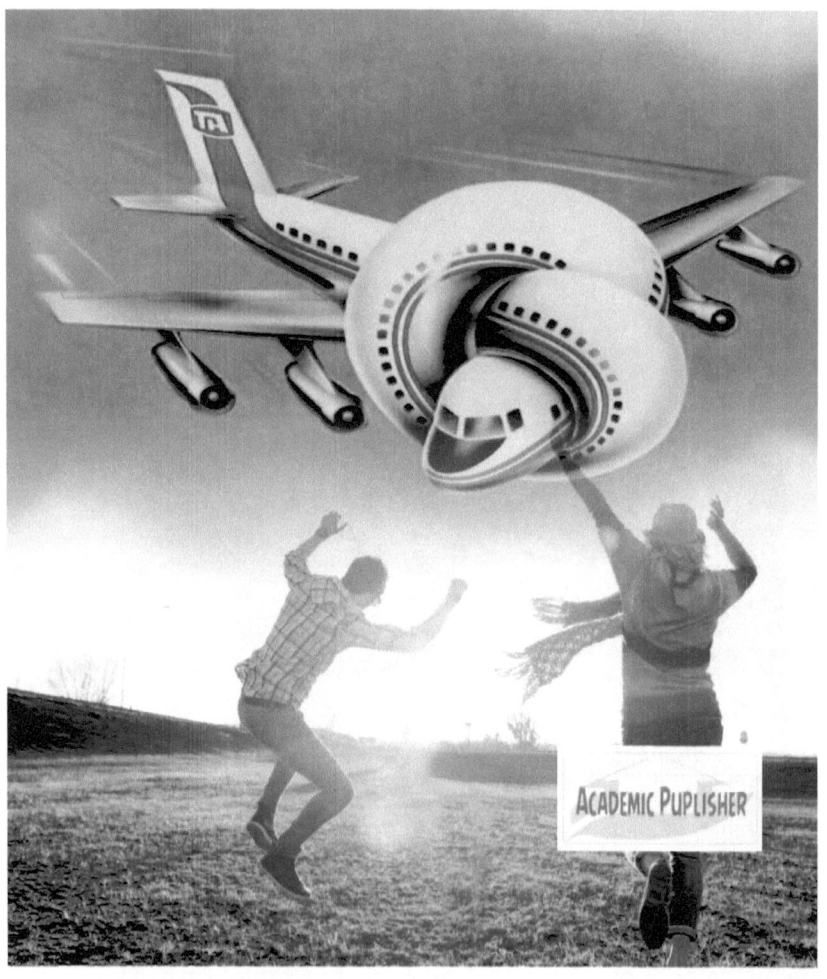

ON THE OTHER HAND : The physical aspect of human harmony with spiritual integration, why?

The integration is a key target in the presence Each asset is seeking integration and within motivation and drive towards integration, logically that fasting produces a healthy integration but the main goal is moral integration. This integration, which achieves the goal of the universe, we refer to access to justice or just society, which achieves the ideal of happiness, Human to rise to the higher level of planned. Figure (2) shows the stages of the divine project. We will discuss this in detail in the following pages.

Chapter 2: SALVATION

First talk

AN INTEGRATION is the primary principle of creatures and the universal essences of beings once for all, but in two levels as:

The first type: Optional integration

The second type: Forced integration

Optional integration respect for human, especially in the intellectual, moral and spiritual side. And the forced integration applies to all physical existence and the Material aspect and physical part of the human.

The law of integration is still at work, not only saving these creatures in their very existence but effecting the progress, and sustenance.

Even now in his providence he is bringing about the assimilation of particulars to universals until he might unite creatures' own voluntary inclination to the more universal natural principle of rational being through the movement of these particular creatures toward well-being, and make them harmonious and self-moving in relation to one another and to the whole universe.[7]

Researcher [7] interested in the subject of the overall integration of the universe and human. It has been discussing this serious matter in terms of religious, but the topic needs to be a wider study as well as to reflect on the ultimate goal of this integration, not only from the religious side but also by the physical and secular trend, especially the Marxist trend and the intellectual side of the capitalist economic.

Fig. 3 showed Classification of intellectual trends of the subject.

ANOTHER THING, what are the limits of this integration? What is the end? What is the usefulness ..?

Is it integrates us happiness? At the individual level or total? for human and for mankind?

Questions produces other questions.. Is there a just future for humankind? Is the fate of the world to the well-being? Is happiness spread throughout us?

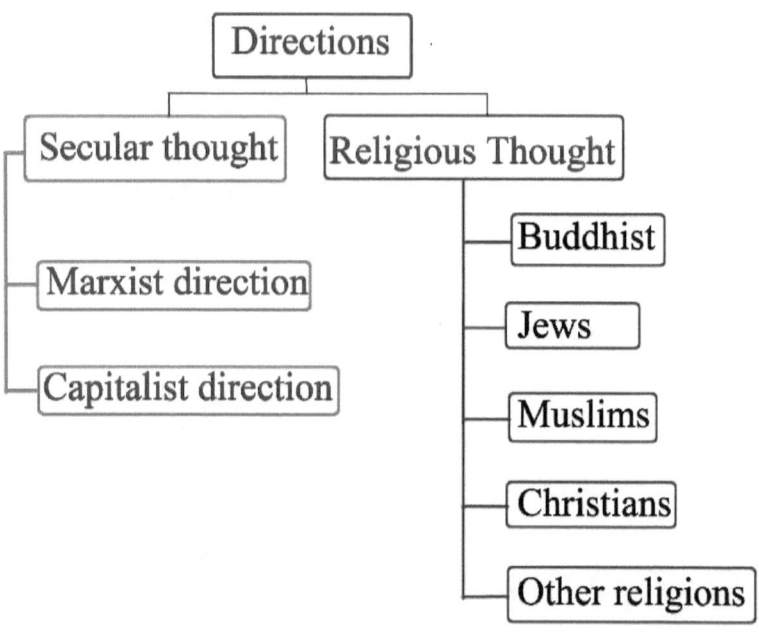

Fig. 3 showed Classification of intellectual trends of the subject.

Marxism And Integration

DEAR READER We are talking about fasting, What is the relationship of that Marxist ideas?

It seems that the talk is about fasting and integration, and the integration is the first goal of fasting. So be the first address for our conversation is integration, as fast as one of the ways in which human reach integration. Marxist thought believes in integration but he does not believe in fasting path of integration.

MARXISTS BELIEVE that the integration gets automatically to humans by the conflict with the other. Marxists believe that integration is the result of the conflict between the classes of society between the working class and the bourgeoisie. The essence of human change depending on social class only and get change if the individual has shifted from (bourgeois) to (factor). Nothing to do with issues of moral and esoteric integration. And the integration of the universe and the community is because of a conflict of opposites or dialectics.

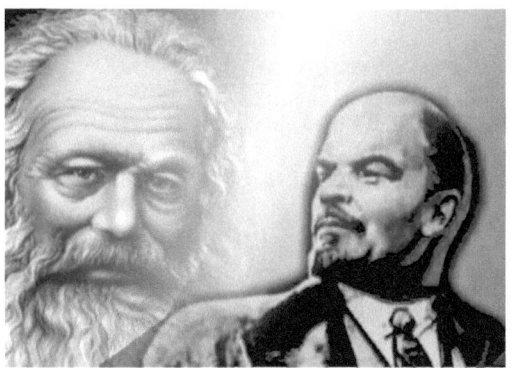

Is There Any Salvation?

We can understand salvation, as the end of human suffering, and the beginning of a new time, is the era of happiness, justice and comfort. The question is: Does this happen ..?

The reader may see this strange question, because he believes that humanity, will stay on this course, suffer problems and injustice. The present conditions all indicate despair.

The human nature of selfishness, sexual or economic or other factor is the cause of this fact, it is the fate of humanity to an end, then, it must be in line with the injustice of human remains to an end, and there is no happy future for us.

This talk is relatively true ..! However, a number of thinkers in the world on the various principles and stripes were able to tracing the future, and to predict the existence of the happy future, and made it clear clues and evidence on it.

For example: If you ask Marxism: Is there a happy future for us ...? They will answer with confidence and reassurance: yes. And if you ask General religions and answered with one voice: Yes, certainly. From this angle will be shared out the search.

Marxism And Salvation

MARXISM INTERESTED in the happy future, based on the general theory developed by the interpretation of history, called Historical Materialism[2], and made its goal happy future for mankind.

So we'll show a detailed presentation of the Marxist views, to see her health, is it has reached introductions demonstrative correct or incorrect, according to the particular methodology for this book known to the people of logic in a manner induction, as we pointed out to it previously.

After Marxism failed, and proved to be the steadfastness of historical materiality to criticism. The question again: Is the prophecy failed, then?! ...

Nope ... there is evidence it can be established. That is the evidence of religion ... which proves the existence of salvation and happy future. That religion could give a good alternative to the Marxist historical materialism, and fills all the historical and social gaps that Marxism tried to fill it, and that did not work.

Answer religions even widely respected ... and he sees it having happy future as a result of human history as a whole, and human existence as a whole as a result of cosmic phenomena and objectives

OF THE PUBLIC. So, happy future is irrelevant to the global goals to herself ... and this will result in universal human an inconclusive future results. Talk will not end when the mere existence of prophecy, as he went Marxism.

Just as religions predicted, this happy future for humanity To demonstrate the existence of a certain commander of the savior of

mankind and the Savior of grievances have problems angle ... has called Islam the Mahdi. The result is the same, the assertion that there happy future. This is the main point of strength.

Hence the author would like, with openness, receive constructive criticism Savior of every critic of the materialists and religious, hoping he could fill in the blanks left by the aspects of human imperfection in his research ... if. Perhaps we reach that conviction to the full main findings.

Salvation In Christian

IN CHRISTIAN THEOLOGY, Jesus is sometimes referred to as a Redeemer. This refers to the salvation he is believed to have accomplished, and is based on the metaphor of redemption, or "buying back". Although the Gospels do not use the title "Redeemer", the word "redemption" is used in several of Paul's letters. Leon Morris says that "Paul uses the concept of redemption primarily to speak of the saving significance of the death of Christ."[8] The English word redemption means 'repurchase' or 'buy back', and in the Old Testament referred to the ransom of slaves (Exodus 21:8).[9] In the New Testament the redemption word group is used to refer both to deliverance from sin and freedom from captivity.[10]

Salvation In Jewish

ONE WRITER say what its content: Salvation is not a Jewish concept, as it implies a focus on the afterlife, which is not significant focus of Judaism. Jews believe that people are supposed to do the best they can at being good. We do this because it is the right thing to do—any personal gain is a side-effect. In fact, focussing on issues of reward and punishment to some extent mitigates the good one is doing by tainting it with selfish motives.

But we do not agree with this view, because we believe that all humanity, general and individual, has defended toward salvation, he forced a formative and defended, not optional ..! But that all assets are seeking to salvation, but it is not the traditional salvation, as in churches and temples, that salvation is a result of human struggle and the struggle for the spiritual and moral integration, it will be up to us happy future.

SALVATION IS ATTAINABLE through the worship of God alone. A person must believe in God and follow His commandments. This is the same message taught by all the Prophets including Moses and Jesus. There is only One worthy of worship. One God, alone without partners, sons, or daughters. Salvation and thus eternal happiness can be achieved by sincere worship.

In addition to this Islam teaches person that human beings are born without sin and are naturally inclined to worship God alone (without any intermediaries). To retain this state of sinlessness humankind must only follow God's commandments and strive to live a righteous life. If one falls into sin, all that is required is sincere repentance followed by seeking God's forgiveness. When a person sins he or she pushes themselves away from the mercy of God, however sincere repentance brings a person back to God.

This understanding of traditional general, the author does not find him expressing the essence of religion and Islam, so I will talk about a new vision in the next chapters of this book.

Salvation in Buddhism

SALVATION IN BUDDHISM follows a different paradigm or template because human evil is not viewed as sin against God or violation of his commands. Human evil is grounded in fundamental ignorance. It is not the simple ignorance of facts, but a blindness to our true nature as passion-ridden beings filled with hate, greed and the delusion of our own goodness. Such ignorance causes the violence and suffering we see in our world perpetrated by humans. We are in bondage to our egos and driven by unknown forces in our subconscious. In Buddhism karma functions as the predisposition to engage in actions whose roots lies beyond the boundaries of our consciousness.

Salvation By Technology

THE BASIC IDEA in this thesis are: Modern science and technology development is the way to deliver human society to the happiness and well-being and especially in the future when science develops more than it is now, and Drjataisal more tests to high levels can ensure them a happy future for all humanity.

How not?!... We see the major outcomes of the science in this day and this age, not only find the reason to respect the technical Victories. If we assume that we passed the major scientific achievements, such as the bombing of maize and rise to the planets and the establishment of electronic brain, If left behind, and we tried to look at the social benefits that science can be achieved is guaranteed for a high level of human happiness and well-being.

So, we have seen much ... there are devices, which invented and continues to invent to overcome the difficulties of home life, and perhaps the most important so far this robot who perform services in all open-mindedness and without tiring !, provides for the family greater efforts. It is also answer the phone and tell the owner of the phone calls taking place during his absence.

IF WE WERE ABLE to join the wonderful results of science to the just and the law of a sound system ... we were able to ensure true luxury grand and happiness, as the scientific results will be distributed that day between human beings equally and without disproportionate unfairness or injustice.

But if we look at the science alone, and we expected him to be an architect for the future happiness with the overthrow of the regime from the view of mind ... it means access to disastrous results harrowing abysmal and prejudice.

Legal Salvation

AFTER THAT it proved the failure of industrial thesis to lead the world, which was based on technological development, and that the important thing is having a good and fair system of law which coordinates society and human affairs, and easy access to their hopes and remove her pain. So the main Commander of mankind for the better is the same law ... which will ensure a future for human beings happy.

The human was and still, going through in its long history and experience of the problems, which are the primary sponsor for the advancement of legal thought. And after the passage of legal thought in two stages:

STEP I: clearly identify the general problems that prevail in society, and to try to understand the full depth and see the understanding of the causes and consequences very carefully.

... If expanded intellectual awareness in the human reality, and understand the problems and sufferings, whenever helped to the legal aspect of farming it.

STEP II: Try depth, in the knowledge of the possible solutions to these problems are offered, and access to effective methods to remove difficulties and overcome obstacles, and then to find well-being and justice in society.

IF LEGAL THINKER, able, to pass both phases, accurately and comprehensively, was able to - inevitably - be up to the development of a just law, which guarantees lasting happiness and well-being.

It still the legal thinking of human beings, in the way of education and integration constantly, from both sides, as a result of social experiments give the accuracy and richness.

And thereby enrich the understanding of jurisprudence ... it is given legal definitions and interpretations are more accurate and comprehensive slowly, whether the one hand, civil or military, or international sanctions laws or personal status law ... or others.

Law in the present era has arrived to supervised graduate ... So it became more accurate humanities. If we may find in it some shortcomings and differences between the thinkers in a number of fields ... the gradual integration of the law, through long experience, is liable to remove these shortcomings and increase the awareness of the legal thinking of those two phases core, which opens to the law a chance gradual access to the realization of real justice, and full belittling human problems.

And where it is not intended, set a certain period of this integration ... it is possible that the law up to that great result, in a future period of eternity, no matter how long.

IF THE LAW arrived to the point of full understanding of justice ... and it can be applied in human society, this is a happy future [promised] in which the well-being and happiness prevail throughout the whole of human society.

However, he can debate this result in spite of its importance, a number of discussions:

DISCUSSION: If we passed the main discussion was the proof in the religious beliefs Research, which is the inability of the human intellect to recognize the real legal interests and the realization of justice ... and therefore he is unable to cover the above two steps, referred to the required and expected to win the full rigor of justice.

It is limited to cover it by divine wisdom, and inspiration behind nature. The human understanding is separated from revelation - as it is imposed on this thesis -, are not able to it in any case. So we will not get salvation legal thought alone.

If we passed that problem, several discussions remained, including the following:

THE FIRST DEBATE: It's hard to imagine that in a possible human legal thought that enriches and integrates constantly, until it reaches the ultimate realization of justice.

THIS IS BECAUSE the legal thinker, whether an individual or a group, shall live in society like any other person, his interests and connections and relationships and economic resources, and so on. It would like in all of this - according to the love of himself - to succeed in all fields, and is ahead of other people.

If legal thinker, with an ideological or political orientation, he was - inevitably - so enthusiastic to his direction, and he would like to win and control over others ... and he would not like losing. In any case, it is a legal person, his composition and direction of social mood, which is impossible for him to depose him from the legal idea ... Whatever the individual tried to take professionalism and objectivity, and impartiality of the selfishness and intolerance ... and the perception of others' interests apart from the interests of the same ... it is a failed and wrong, because of no sense pushing it, involuntarily, as well as public pressure and the circumstances, and his past, that imposes on himelf from what he knows and does not know.

THE SECOND DEBATE: that the legal theory, no matter escalated and integrated, not only to ensure the rule of happiness and justice among the people ... but, it is necessary to take the path to the application in the world of life, to be able to come to fruition mature appetite.

Nor can any human law that an individual tracks always, and everywhere, to ensure the full application of paragraphs and clauses in

All The Time. It is impossible to state with all its dominance and prestige and its institutions, to ensure that.

If possible, sometimes, you can not always ... While he could always, in an individual or a particular group, you will not be in all the people. As would be unable to apply the law of the General him and convinced him to accept the heart. But the law will be applied to the extent required by the power of the hand, and the personal interests of individuals on the other hand ... by paying themselves punishment, or obtain it something of interest.

Chapter 3: New Vision

AT THE OUTSET, it is worth us to learn about the nature of human and reality, because materialist thinking dominated our culture, and we became look at the humans that they are only physical assets, and this is not true. Human is material and moral and spiritual.

It could be argued that the moral side of man is divided into three sections:

First: the spiritual section.

Second, the psychological or soul section.

Third: the mental section. Figure (2) a possible representation of this thesis.

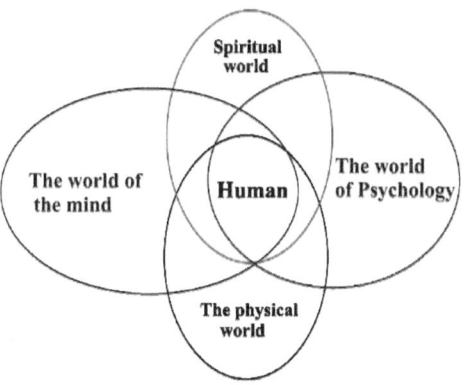

Figure (2) a possible representation of this thesis.

The World Of The Mind

THERE ARE TWO possibilities for the relationship of the physical part with the moral parts; The first possibility: that the portions overlapping with each other in our world, and the second possibility that the mind, spirit and soul, they are not here, in our world, but they exist in their world, outside the physical world. Figure(3) illustrates the second possibility.

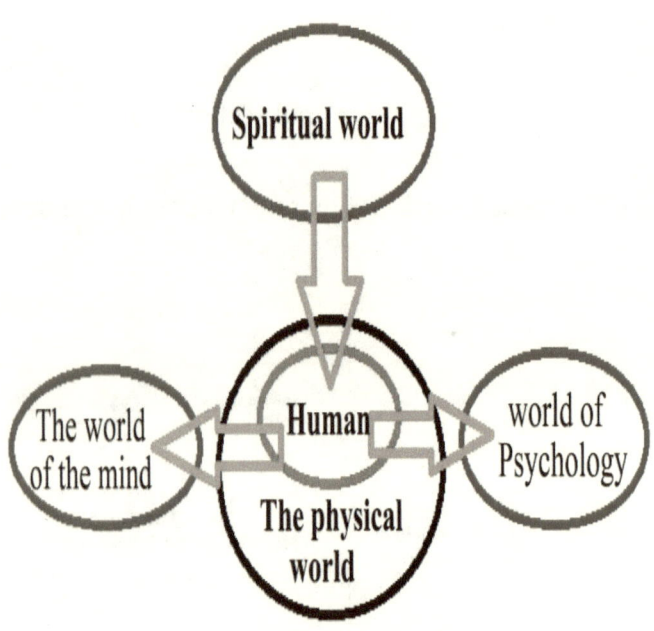

Figure(3) illustrates the second possibility.

Self-Management

SO HUMAN BEINGS needs to be integration and development in the rest of the other parts, not enough physical integration. We also need to rearrange the relationship between our parts, and better to have the mind and spirit is stronger than the body and the soul.

We could say: that the body responsible for self-management and animal requirements, while Spirit is interested in conjunction occult powers, and is interested in mind the overall administration of material and moral parts.

And joyful thing, the divine law imposes development and integration. Despite these inevitable it is not clear to us, because short of our lives, but it is clear in the long human life.

This fact is heartening, it is managed by the general planning for the development of the universe and humanity, and we can call it common law to raise the universe and humanity[3]. And I try in this book to offer early stages of this thesis, new vision, and may be strange in the

---

3a concept that I read it for the first time, in the books of the Iraqi thinker Alsadr or Muhammed alsader (1943-1999). His book named Encyclopedia of Imam Mahdi.

eyes of dear reader, because we are talking out of tune, and against the traditionally accepted.

The Human System

THE NEW THING that we are saying: that the human system integration needs for a fair judgment, and this inevitably will be achieved, in accordance with divine law overall, this is not a religious radical. On the contrary, because the current religious reality is crippling the Divine for the project. The divine plan does not differentiate between humans and another, and rejects racism and violence, but seeks for a stable situation in which integrates human until it reaches the maximum degree of integration, which is salvation, because humans will open on the metaphysical vision of the world, live master of the existence of the whole.

Figure below, it represents the thesis that: The worlds vary in intensity, as are voices differ in their frequencies, so you hear certain frequencies, and can not hear frequencies that are all around us, but with certain modes, or special abilities. The worlds exist around us, overlapping them, because of their different densities. The moral integrity of humankind, may be able to open up to other worlds, and this explains the reason for its existence in the universe. Is likely to be the mind is least intense, because he has the mind of man, not an animal, while Spirit found in most of the assets. Note that with the mind in the animal is limited, not up to the level of the human mind

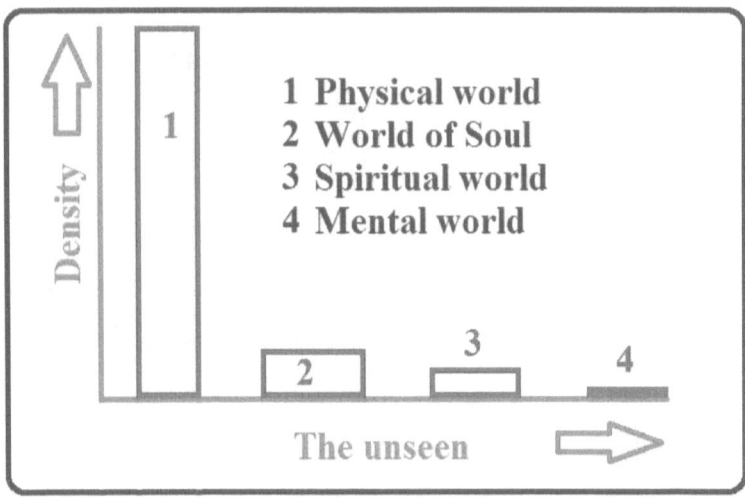

Speech above, it is an opinion only, although there are sources to it, but we do not see these worlds, only in a dream, or we heard about it from some body, who have returned to our world after the death. The aim of this thesis is to understand the relationship of the integration of human fate and future.

Final word:

FROM HERE we understand the importance of fasting, because he is one of integration tools needed by the divine project, in spite of attempts to offer a better perception of this thesis, but I acknowledged that the current completeness, and I promise to dear reader, I am trying to write better than this, do not hesitate to communicate, to take advantage of feedback in providing the best of this production. The last thing, I say that the whole intellectual trends, are human attempts, some of which complements the others, and Marxism and secular, are attempt to understand the presence, for the sake of integration, but they focused on the physical aspect, and neglected the most important aspects in humans.

Chapter 4: Christianity and salvation

The Birth Of Jesus

THE IDEA OF SALVATION have closely Christian thought, so this chapter has been added to this book, in the final moments, for the fulfillment of the idea of salvation and historical introductions, then linked to the divine project. An analysis was obtained by us for this historical review, we hope that the reader tolerate us, because we're trying to get to the truth impartially, as much as possible.

We knew enough idea of the conditions that sent through Jesus Christ the son of Mary, was the ruling power strong dictatorship, social atmosphere of the state engaging obstinate, religious Jewish atmosphere based on the deviation and intolerance, and the priests twisting the law. Though they were waiting for a new reformer, but they expected to be a reformer of the Jews, the guarantor of all that they aspire of ambitions.

CHRIST WAS BORN without a father, in order to several conclusions:

First result: Notice of society, that this newborn important people of the divine, and not a layman like all other people.

The second conclusion: that this miracle evidence of the purity of Mary and purity.

THIRD CONCLUSION: that this miracle sign of his prophethood and high stature in the divine project.

His mother was a devout and conservative family, but this is not enough to prove her innocence in front of the clergy - then - so it got a significant miracle, proved the prophecy of Jesus and His Holiness, as well as the innocence of his mother, that miracle is: his early pronunciation, that he spoke in a cradle, in the first month of his birth.

The evidence uttered by the prophets - who they came after him - for the prophecy of Jesus, which is explained the importance of Jesus and his call for a global, the Bible was not enough to prove the new religion of Jesus. He did not say the universality of his call, and did not know about the law of social and economic integrated. Hence can not be for Christians to look to him more than a prophet of the Prophets of Israel, a continuation of the law of Moses, peace be upon him came, like Isaiah and Jeremiah and Daniel.

But the Divine planning to support the religion of Jesus, by the prophets after him, and proved to us his new religion, and show us the future role of Jesus in human salvation and the establishment of a just social system, and we hope to have it soon, after the return of Jesus to the world.

We await the day of salvation, led by Christ, is supposed to be - we - the level of responsibility, we leave delusions and courtesies, and obey Allah and His Messenger, and Allah's Messenger, according to

The Evidence and the correct sources, after research and investigation by us all.

And we shall continue spiritually with God, by fasting, because it raises the barriers between us and God, we do not need it formality, but internally and mystically by fasting, and provides us with a good opportunity to pray and request divine help, down to the right way. Because the person is responsible for obedience in accordance with the true and correct to the divine orders.

The arrest and killing of Christ

NECESSARY TO EXPOSURE to the incident of the arrest of Christ and try to kill him. Christ has been harmed by a violent priests, and the Romanian government. As well as he had been betrayed by one of his disciples, Judas Iscariot, who guided authorities to the place of Jesus, after the rule of the Jewish Council of wasting his blood.

There is no need to go into details of incidents, because it is available to the reader in its sources, but it is important that the death of Christ are two possibilities:

First thesis: that he died crucified, as people die crucified, after the conspiracy hatched against him succeeded.

It seems that the Jews and the Christians agree on the amount of the thesis, but the Christians say - according to the Gospels - that Christ came back into the world again - after the killing - and then ascended to heaven in front of his students.

The second thesis: that Christ did not die like all other people, but the Almighty - accidentally marvelous - Christ saved from this plot, and raised him. So he has ascended to heaven without dying.

And now we want the preference treatise on the other. But it is important to harmonize the one with the divine plan.

IT SEEMS THAT the first thesis, more logical, because a failed society spiritually and morally, it may cause to kill him. But the appearance of Christ after three days, it is possible reason, but there was no evidence, according to extrapolate texts and checked by the researcher. It seems - historically - that people who say the vision of Christ - after three days - the ones who have strayed from Christianity after Christ. So, they are unreliable in the news for this vision. In addition to that the idea faced strong cash by Christians modernists, as Charles Jnneber in his book; Christian .. origins and evolution.

By the second thesis, we can look to the two levels:

First level: the boarding accident - marvelous - imposed from outside the human range. So, the reality is part of the overall planning divine, not human planning. Therefore, we are not responsible for the statement of the philosophy of it, because many of the cosmic planning points, still invisible to the human mind.

The second level: that in spite of the fact that boarding a miracle, but it is not without its link to humanity, as predicted return of Christ to the world in the future, in order to participate in the overall planning of the Divine Project.

Mention may be made to two points:

First:

THE SECOND THESIS involved with the Gospels in the idea of Christ's ascension in his spirit and his body to heaven. and diverge with it, why.? because the Gospels tell of his death first and then carrying out of his grave, and his ascension to heaven, while the second thesis says his ascension to heaven from the world of life directly.

Two:

IF WE DID NOT TAKE the second thesis, it does not mean that we be binding proposals to reject the idea of returning to the world again. But it remains possible !!, everything in it that he died like all other people, then live to the world again. If ratified say re-entry of Christ, and it was necessary for the success of the state of right and future government, with the presumption of sincerity first thesis, the commitment with his life after death is necessary, in order to ensure the success of the divine project.

It seems that the return of Jesus Christ has become necessary, in accordance with the divine plan. Why..?

Christians feel that they became - gradually - that contemporary Christian faith in all its forms, do not represent Jesus Christ. And from it - my hand - These two books are: Christ is not a Christian] to Bernard Shaw, and Christian origins and evolution] Charles Junbaar. Perhaps the books and other ideas as well.

What I care about this talk, it is the fact that a statement of salvation, which is linked with relapsing Christ and to achieve justice in the human. And it is not intended to offend any religion or orientation, but the free search humanitarian and moral necessity.

I will try to expand on this subject at the end chance, coming edition, or a new book, Greetings to you, my friend, reader, and you can send me your feedback, I welcome them to my mail:

drnadhim@gmail.com

Note that the book was printed two types, economic copy and a normal copy, digital copy.

HISTORICAL MATERIALISM is a methodological approach to the study of human societies and their development over time and was first articulated by Karl Marx (1818–1883) as the materialist conception of history. It is principally a theory of history according to which the material conditions of a society's mode of production (its way of producing and reproducing the means of human existence or, in Marxist terms, the union of its productive capacity and social relations of production) fundamentally determine its organization and development. https://en.wikipedia.org

FASTING:

The verb; (1) fast used without object to abstain from all food, to eat only sparingly or of certain kinds of food, especially as a religious observance. (2) verb used with object to cause to abstain entirely from or limit food; put on a fast: to fast a patient for a day before surgery.

The noun; an abstinence from food, or a limiting of one's food, especially when voluntary and as a religious observance; fasting.

http://www.dictionary.com/

MORAL INTEGRATION:

Moral integration is the virtue of doing good. This requires determining what the right thing to do is, and then doing exactly that. Moral integration unites the various

virtues and motivates your good actions. The virtues are mere abstractions until they are applied and acted upon, and moral integration prepares us for that action.

https://en.wikiversity.org/

LOGIC INDUCTION:

argument." Main source: Induction Def. "the derivation of general principles from specific instances" is called induction.

An inductive logic:

An inductive logic is a system of evidential support that extends deductive logic to less-than-certain inferences. For valid deductive arguments the premises logically entail the conclusion, where the entailment means that the truth of the premises provides a guarantee of the truth of the conclusion. Similarly, in a good inductive argument the premises should provide some degree of support for the conclusion, where such support means that the truth of the premises indicates with some degree of strength that the conclusion is true. Presumably, if the logic of good inductive arguments is to be of any real value, the measure of support it articulates should meet special conditions.

References

[1] Nicholas F. Gier (2004). The Virtue of Nonviolence: From Gautama to Gandhi. SUNY Press. p. 222. ISBN 978-0-7914-5949-2.

[2] Stedman's medical dictionary (28th ed.). Philadelphia: Lippincott Williams & Wilkins. 2006. ISBN 978-0-7817-3390-8.

[3] Hawton K, van Heeringen K (April 2009). "Suicide". Lancet 373 (9672): 1372–81. doi:10.1016/S0140-6736(09)60372-X. PMID 19376453.

[4] "Suicide Fact sheet N°398". WHO. August 2015. Retrieved 3 March 2016.

[5] Bottino, SM; Bottino, CM; Regina, CG; Correia, AV; Ribeiro, WS (March 2015). "Cyberbullying and adolescent mental health: systematic review.". Cadernos de saude publica 31 (3): 463–75. doi:10.1590/0102-311x00036114. PMID 25859714.

[6] Sakinofsky, I (June 2007). "The current evidence base for the clinical care of suicidal patients: strengths and weaknesses". Canadian Journal of Psychiatry 52 (6 Suppl 1): 7S–20S. PMID 17824349.

[7] Andrea Elizabeth, "On God's Preservation and Integration of the Universe".

https://bloggingsbetter.wordpress.com

[8]   Borgen, Peder. Early Christianity and Hellenistic Judaism. Edinburgh: T & T Clark Publishing. 1996.

[9] Brown, Raymond. An Introduction to the New Testament. New York: Doubleday. 1997.

[10] Dunn, J. D. G.. Christology in the Making. London: SCM Press. 1989.

[11] Free Encyclopedia.

https://en.wikipedia.org

[12] Marxists internet Archive .

https://www.marxists.org/

[13] Alsadr, Mohummed, Encyclopedia of Imam Mahdi, Iraq, Najaf, body legacy of the martyr Sadr.2012.

[14] Alsadr, Mohummed, Jurisprudence ethics, Iraq, Najaf, body legacy of the martyr Sadr.2012.

[15] Alsadr, Mohummed, Beyond the jurisprudence, Iraq, Najaf, body legacy of the martyr Sadr.2012.

[16] Daniel Cobb, Derek Olsen (ed.). Saint Augustine's Prayer Book. pp. 4–5.

[17] Kallistos (Ware), Bishop; Mary, Mother (1978). The Lenten Triodion. South Canaan PA: St. Tikhon's Seminary Press (published 2002). pp. 35ff. ISBN 1-878997-51-3.

[18] Kallistos (Ware), Bishop (1964). The Orthodox Church. London: Penguin Books. pp. 75–77, 306ff. ISBN 0-14-020592-6.

[19] Gregory Palamas, Letter 234, I (Migne, Patrologia Graecae, 1361C)

[20] "Old Orthodox Prayer Book" (2nd ed.). Erie PA: Russian Orthodox Church of the Nativity of Christ (Old Rite). 2001: 349ff.

[21] "August 1991". Stjamesok.org. Retrieved 2016-01-11.

[22] "John Wesley and Spiritual Disciplines-- The Works of Piety". The United Methodist Church. 2012. Retrieved 5 April 2014.

[23 Beard, Steve (30 January 2012). "The spiritual discipline of fasting". Good News Magazine (United Methodist Church).

[24] Abraham, William J.; Kirby, James E. (2009-09-24). The Oxford Handbook of Methodist Studies. Oxford University Press. pp. 257–. ISBN 978-0-19-160743-1.

[25] Grumett, David and Rachel Muers. 2010. Theology on the menu: asceticism, meat and Christian diet. P.55

[26] Albala, Ken. 2003. Food in early modern Europe. P.200

[27] J. Gordon Melton. Encyclopedia of Protestantism. P.219-220

[28] Poole, Kristen (2006-03-30). Radical Religion from Shakespeare to Milton: Figures of Nonconformity in Early Modern England. Cambridge University Press. ISBN 978-0-521-02544-7.

[29] Archived November 2, 2009, at the Wayback Machine.

[30] What is the holiest season of the Church Year?. Retrieved 2010-02-03. Archived copy at the Internet Archive

[31] An explanation of Luther's Small Catechism: The Sacrament of the Eucharist, section IV: Who receives the Sacrament worthily? (LCMS). Retrieved 2009-10-15.

[32] Wallis, Arthur, God's Chosen Fast, Christian Literature Crusade (June 1986)

[33] Johnson, William, The Fasting Movement, Bethesda Books, 2003

[34] Shelton, Herbert, The Science and Fine Art of Fasting, American Natural Hygiene Society, Incorporate; 5th edition (August 1978)

[35] "Neurodegenerative Diseases and Fasting". Antiaging-europe.com. Retrieved 2010-10-18.

[36] Riley M. Lorimer. "Where Do Fast Offerings Go? - New Era May 2008 – new-era". Lds.org. Retrieved 2016-01-11.

[37] Gordon B. Hinckley. "The State of the Church – Ensign May 1991 – ensign". Lds.org. Retrieved 2016-01-11.

[38] "First Presidency Letter: Testimonies in Fast and Testimony Meeting – Church News and Events". Lds.org. Retrieved 2016-01-11.

[39] "Shravan Month, Shravan Maas, Sawan Mahina 2015". Rudraksha Ratna. Retrieved 2016-01-11.

[40] "The Mahabharata, Book 13: Anusasana Parva: Section CIII". www.sacred-texts.com. Retrieved 2015-10-19.

[41] "The Mahabharata, Book 13: Anusasana Parva: Section CIX". www.sacred-texts.com. Retrieved 2015-10-19.

[42] "The Mahabharata, Book 13: Anusasana Parva: Section CVI". www.sacred-texts.com. Retrieved 2015-10-19.

[43] "Official Ramadan 2014 website". Ramadan.co.uk. Retrieved 2016-01-11.

[44] Ismail Kamus (1993). Hidup Bertaqwa (2nd ed.). Kuala Lumpur: At Tafkir Enterprise. ISBN 983-99902-0-9.

[45] Prero, Yehuda. "The Fast of the Tenth of Teves, "Asara B'Teves"". Project Genesis. Retrieved August 1, 2010.

[46] Posner, Menachem. "Why fast after dropping a Torah scroll or tefillin? - Questions & Answers". Chabad.org. Retrieved 2016-01-

[47] Lampronti, Paḥad Yiẓḥaḳ, Berlin, 1887;

[48] W. R. Smith, Rel. of Sem. London, 1894;

[49] Monteflore, Hibbert Lectures, London, 1897;

[50] Oehler, Theologie des Alten Testaments, Stuttgart, 1891;

[51] Dembitz, Jewish Services in Synagogue and Home, Philadelphia, 1898.

[52] Shaw, R. (2008)Beyond the Fields: Cesar Chavez, the UFW, and the struggle for justice in the 21st century University of California Press, p.92

[53] Espinosa, G. Garcia, M Mexican American Religions:Spirituality activism and culture(2008) Duke University Press, p 108

[54] Shaw, R. (2008)Beyond the Fields: Cesar Chavez, the UFW, and the struggle for justice in the 21st century University of California Press, p.93

[55] Smith, Peter (2000). "fasting". A concise encyclopedia of the Bahá'í Faith. Oxford: Oneworld Publications. p. 157. ISBN 1-85168-184-1.

[56] Effendi, Shoghi (1973). Directives from the Guardian. Hawaii Bahá'í Publishing Trust. p. 28.

[57] "The Buddhist Monk's Discipline: Some Points Explained for Laypeople". Accesstoinsight.org. 2010-08-23. Retrieved 2010-10-18.

[58] "Kitagiri Sutta-Majjhima Nikaya". Urbandharma.org. Retrieved 2011-03-12.

[59] b Harderwijk, Rudy (2011-02-06). "The Eight Mahayana Precepts". Viewonbuddhism.org. Retrieved 2011-03-12.

[60] "Nyung Ne". Drepung.org. Retrieved 2011-03-12.

[61] "Nyungne Retreat with Lama Dudjom Dorjee". Ktcdallas.org. Retrieved 2011-03-12.

[62] Ph.D, Randi Fredricks (2012-12-20). Fasting: An Exceptional Human Experience. AuthorHouse. ISBN 978-1-4817-2379-4.

[63] http://www.allaboutprayer.org/

[64] http://www.ihopkc.org/

[65] http://biblia.com/

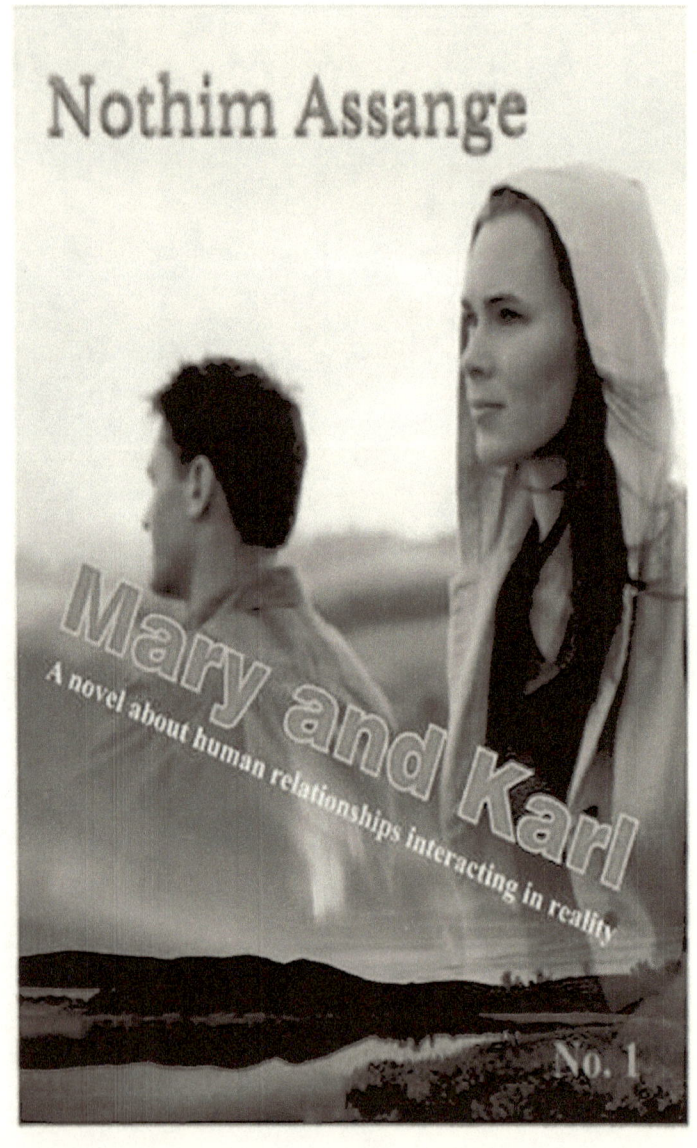

Spiritual integration:

How to develop personal powers

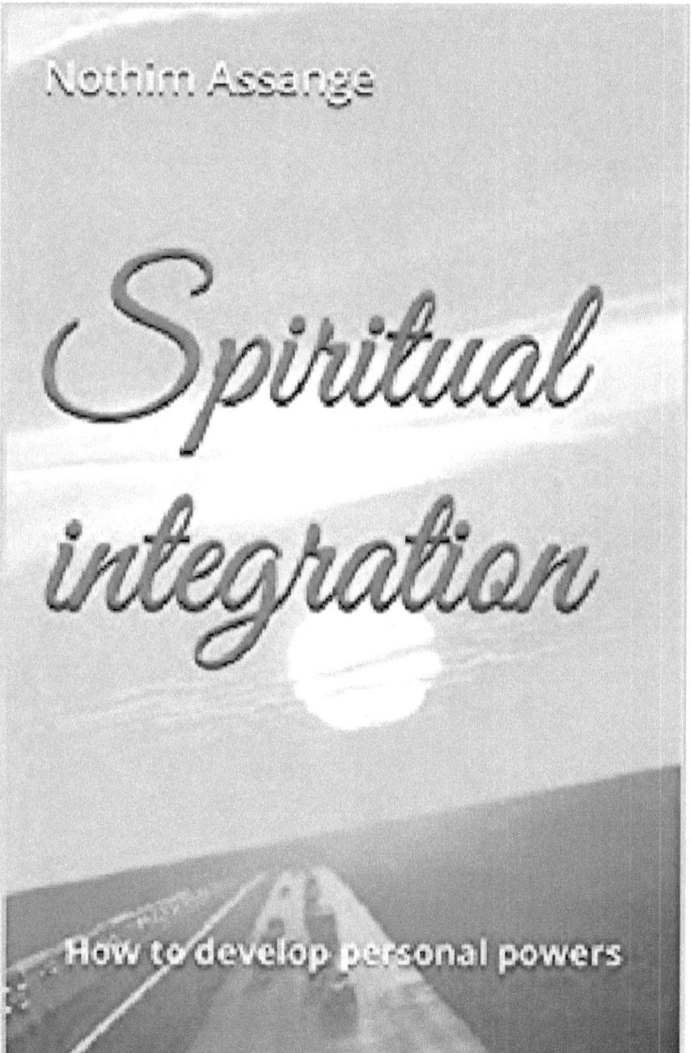

Key to kid

Personal experience may benefit

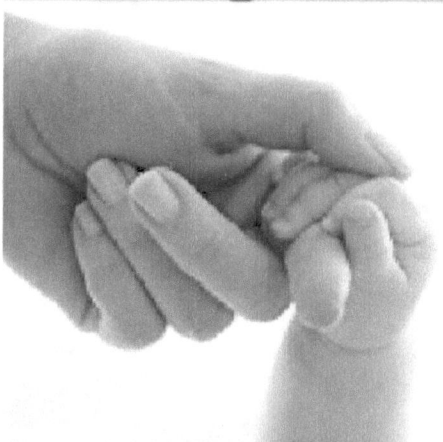

Key to kid

How I was able to
realize my dream ..?

Nothim Assange

FASTING AND SAVLATION

Note:

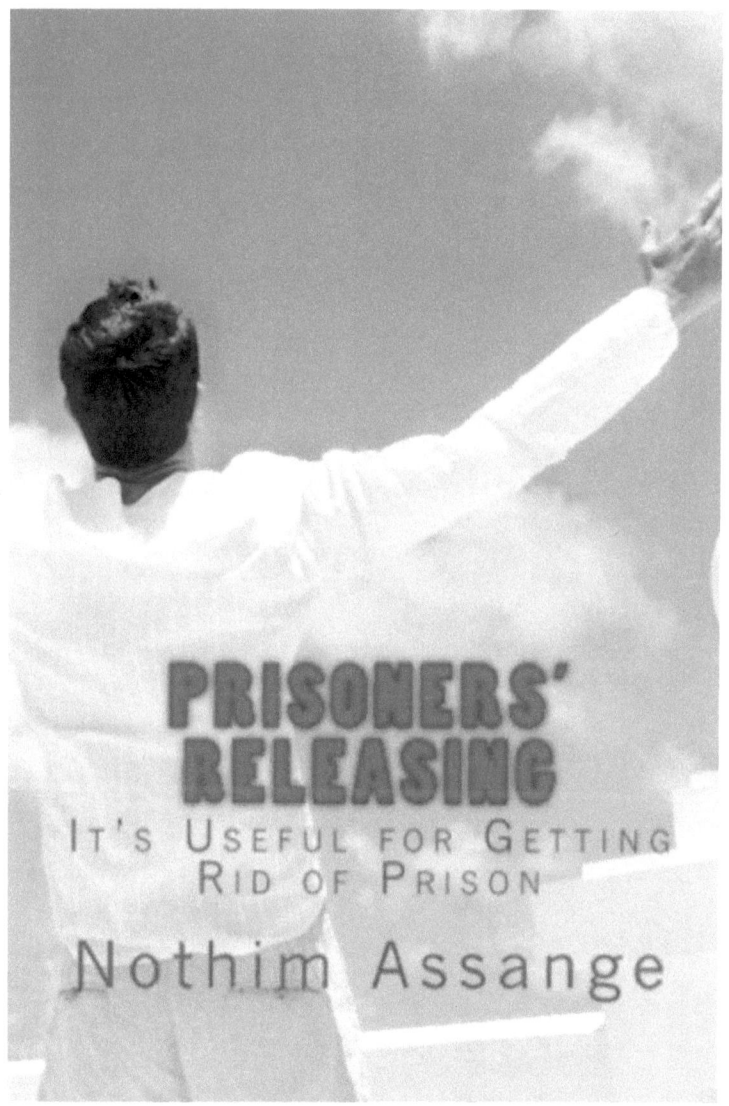

Note: